Maharishi Mahesh Yogi's

Transcendental Meditation

**A New Introduction to Maharishi's Easy, Effective
and Scientifically Proven Technique for
Promoting Better Health, Unfolding Your
Creative Potential—and Creating Peace
in the World**

by Robert Roth

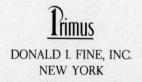

Primus

DONALD I. FINE, INC.
NEW YORK

"I consider myself a very practical person. I am president of a small chemical manufacturing firm. I have a wonderful wife and two great children. And I am concerned about the community that I live in.

"I have been practicing Transcendental Meditation for several years. It gives me more hours to my day and more energy and effectiveness in each hour.

"I wouldn't miss it for the world."

R.W. Montgomery
President
H.A. Montgomery Company
Detroit

"As a cardiologist I work 12- to 16-hour days—and much of it is under emergency conditions. I am continually on call and continually on the go.

"TM gives me the deep rest, mental alertness, and energy boost that I need to meet the constant pressures of my work.

"For this I find 20 minutes of TM more effective than several hours of relaxation or exercise."

James Williams, M.D.
Cardiologist
Austin

"TM is a wonderful technique. It enables you to settle down and become strong within yourself. It also helps to give you the energy, intelligence, and ability to succeed at whatever you do.

"Since beginning TM, I have achieved many of the goals I set for myself, including that of becoming a successful high school student. Now I intend to accomplish much, much more in my life."

Alicia Isen, 17
High School Senior
Fairfield, Iowa

Library of Congress Catalogue Card Number: 87-14568
ISBN: 1-55611-085-5
Manufactured in the United States of America
10 9 8 7 6 5 4 3 2 1

Library of Congress Cataloging-in-Publication Data
Roth, Robert, 1950-
Transcendental Meditation.
"A new introduction to Maharishi's easy,
effective and scientifically proven technique for promoting
better health, unfolding your creative potential—
and creating peace in the world."

1. Transcendental Meditation
I. Title
BF637.T68R68   1987   158'.12   87-14568
ISBN 1-55611-085-5

Printed in the United States of America

Transcendental Meditation® and TM-Sidhi® are service marks of WPEC-US. Maharishi and Maharishi Technology of the Unified Field are the service marks of Maharishi International University.

Table of Contents

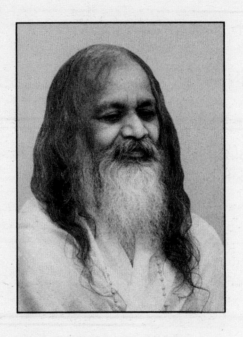

MAHARISHI MAHESH YOGI

Founder of the
Transcendental Meditation
and TM-Sidhi Program and the
Maharishi Technology of the Unified Field

Introduction

On January 30, 1959, Maharishi Mahesh Yogi arrived at San Francisco International Airport. It was his first visit to the United States and the second continent on his global tour to introduce his Transcendental Meditation (TM) technique to the world.

The *San Francisco Chronicle* published an article covering Maharishi's first TM lecture in the city. Several hundred people attended Maharishi's lectures; many learned the technique.

In those early days there were no other TM teachers, no other TM lecturers, no TM organization, no TM centers. After San Francisco, Maharishi spent several months in Los Angeles, then on to New York. And from New York to London, Germany, Greece, and on around the world.

The TM movement started simply and grew steadily. Then, suddenly, with the first published scientific research on the technique, TM dawned in world consciousness.

The first study on TM was conducted at the University of California at Los Angeles in 1968 by physiologist Robert Keith Wallace. His thesis,"The

Physiological Effects of Transcendental Meditation: A Proposed Fourth Major State of Consciousness," earned him his Ph.D. and was published in the journal, *Science*. It also inspired a huge wave of scientific interest into the effects of TM.

By 1975 Transcendental Meditation was a household word.

And today?

Over three million people worldwide—including one million people in the United States—from every profession, age, educational background, and religion practice TM. And the number keeps growing.

There are over 1,500 TM centers established in major cities in 100 countries throughout the world teaching TM under the auspices of non-profit, educational organizations.

TM has been learned by over 6,000 medical doctors in the U.S. and by thousands of executives, managers, and employees of large and small companies throughout the United States and the world.

Housewives practice TM. So do attorneys, computer programmers, teachers, students, salesclerks, clergy, professional athletes, factory workers, architects, airline pilots, electricians, chefs, and artists.

Why?

TM is easy to learn. Anyone can practice it. And it works.

During the past 18 years, over 350 scientific research studies have been conducted on the effects of the TM technique at 160 universities and research institutions in 27 countries. The studies—many of which have been published in leading scientific journals—have shown that the TM program:

- reduces stress
- improves memory and learning ability
- increases energy
- increases inner calm
- reduces insomnia
- increases happiness and self-esteem
- reduces anxiety and depression
- improves relationships
- improves health
- promotes a younger biological age

Since Maharishi first began teaching the TM technique 30 years ago, modern science has made major breakthroughs in understanding how nature functions. Recently, scientists have glimpsed the deepest level of nature's functioning—the unified field of natural law—which is the source of the unlimited creative potential displayed throughout the universe.

As we'll see in this book, the unlimited potential found deep within human consciousness and the unlimited potential found at the level of the unified field are not different; they are the same.

Transcendental Meditation is a simple, effective technique that enlivens this source of unlimited potential in daily life. It enriches all areas of life, just as watering the root of a plant brings nourishment to all parts of the plant.

This book has been written to provide you with a brief and complete introduction to the TM program. It is an introduction to a technique that can change your life, for good.

I hope you enjoy it.

Robert Roth

CHAPTER 1

TM at a Glance

Christine Riegel, 36, is a speech therapist and the mother of five children, ages two to eight. She and her husband, Arthur, an account executive with an employee search firm, live in Corte Madera, a small town north of San Francisco

As with most families, the Riegels' day starts early—6:00 a.m.—and often ends 16 to 18 hours later. There are the older children to get off to school and the younger ones to take care of. And Arthur leaves for work at 7:30 a.m.

Both Christine and Arthur have been practicing TM for several years. They meditate for 20 minutes in the morning before the children wake up, and again in the afternoon—Christine at home before preparing dinner and Arthur at home after work.

"With our schedule and five children, TM is vital," Christine says. Arthur adds: "I find that I have much more energy after practicing TM in the morning. My mind is clearer and more organized. And I find that these benefits last throughout the entire day."

Transcendental Meditation

What is Transcendental Meditation, exactly?
(And what is it not?)
What are the benefits? How does it work?
And what do medical doctors, business leaders, and clergy say about it?

The first thing to know about TM is that it is easy to learn, and it's easy and enjoyable to practice. Second, the scientific research shows that the benefits can be seen immediately and accumulate over time. Third, TM is simple to understand.

What TM Is

Transcendental Meditation is a simple, natural, effortless, easily learned mental technique practiced for 15-20 minutes twice daily sitting comfortably with the eyes closed.

simple—TM is not complicated.

natural—there is no manipulation and no suggestion involved.

effortless—TM is easy to practice and requires no concentration or control.

easily learned—anyone beginning from age 10 can learn TM without any difficulty.

mental technique—it involves no physical exercises, postures, or procedures.

practiced for 15-20 minutes twice daily—TM is practiced once in the morning before breakfast, to start the day with alertness and dynamism.

And once in the afternoon before dinner, to eliminate the stress of the day and prepare for an enjoyable evening and a good night's sleep.

sitting comfortably—there are no awkward positions necessary to practice TM. It can be practiced anywhere—while you're riding the train to work, in a plane, even in a car parked at a freeway rest stop. But it is usually practiced in the comfort of your own home.

What Happens During the TM Technique

During the TM technique the mind settles down to a silent, yet fully awake state of awareness. At the same time the body gains a unique and profound state of rest and relaxation.

To understand this experience, first we'll take an example of its opposite—

It's Friday at 2:00 p.m. It has been a frenetic day, a long week. And it's not over yet.

Late for an appointment, you race to your car only to discover that you've forgotten the keys. Then having found your keys, you battle traffic and finally make it to your appointment—only to realize that you've left behind some important papers.

Your mind is racing, excited. This, needless to say, is a more excited state of the mind.

On the other hand—

It's Sunday afternoon and you're heading home from a weekend vacation—refreshed and rested. You begin to think of ways to improve things at work and at home.

They are good, practical ideas. Your mind is calm, creative, alert. You feel happy. This is a more settled state of the mind.

Both of these experiences—of greater and of lesser excitation of mind and body—are familiar to us. Now what does TM do?

TM allows the mind to settle down to its own silent, "self-referral" state of awareness where the mind is calm, collected, yet fully expanded, fully awake.

This state is the simplest form of human awareness. It is pure consciousness, a state where consciousness is open only to itself—open to its own full potential. And, as we'll see in the next chapter, it is the unified field of natural law, which modern quantum physics describes as the source of the infinite creativity and intelligence of nature.

This settled state of awareness is completely natural to the mind. It has always been there. It was there ten years ago, it's there right now, and it'll be there tomorrow. Only it has been lost from experience, lost from use, because of the constant noise and excitations of daily living.

TM opens the awareness to pure consciousness easily, effortlessly, and enjoyably—for everyone. At the same time, extensive scientific research has shown that while the mind settles down during TM, the body gains a unique and profound state of rest and relaxation.

Benefits of the TM Technique

This deep rest provided by TM eliminates the build-up of stress and tension, and provides the basis for more dynamic and rewarding activity. TM, therefore, is practiced as a preparation for daily activity and not as an end in itself.

Rest eliminates stress. And the deeper the rest, the better. The rest gained during a night's sleep is sufficient to eliminate some of the stress and fatigue resulting from a full day of activity. But obviously a night's sleep, no matter how deep, isn't enough. We may feel better the next morning, but all too often we don't feel completely refreshed, completely renewed.

So we may exercise to help cope with stress. We play tennis, work out at the gym, take an evening stroll. We may listen to soothing music, read a good book, knit a sweater, or go on a fishing trip.

But something is missing. Despite our best efforts, stress clings to the nervous system and builds up day after day, year after year. Butterflies in the stomach from pre-exam nerves at age 16 can turn into stomach ulcers, high blood pressure, or premature aging from too much worry at age 40.

What is missing? Very deep rest.

Recreation, or even a vacation, may be relaxing but they do not provide the deep rest necessary to eliminate stress. Because of this the benefits are short-lived.

(Recall your first day back at work after a week-long vacation. Within a few hours it feels like you never left.)

What is the solution?

TM.

Eliminating Deep Stress

Why? Because it provides very deep rest, which is exactly what the body needs to eliminate the very deep stress that sleep or a vacation never touches. In one stroke of TM the mind and body are rejuvenated. Then you can play tennis, read a book, work in the garden, or go fishing because you enjoy it, and not because you are trying to cope with an ever-increasing amount of stress in life.

In the past, meditation has been considered the concern of recluses. For people with families and jobs meditation, at its best, was seen as a momentary refuge from the demands of living; at its worst, an escape from life.

TM is neither. It is a practical technique for dynamic, intelligent, rewarding activity. It is a technique to develop the full potential of mind and body—the basis for success and satisfaction in life.

What TM Is Not

TM is not a religion, a philosophy, or a lifestyle. Nor does it involve any codes of conduct or moral training, a value system, belief, or worship.

TM is not a religion—it's a technique. People of all religions, including clergy, practice TM. It supports all religions because it releases stress and purifies the mind, body, and emotions of the person who practices it.

TM is not a philosophy—it's a simple, mechanical technique. Turning on a night light is a technique, not a philosophy. Using a lever to move a large rock is a technique, not a philosophy. And TM is a scientific technique because it is universally applicable, repeatable, and verifiable by anyone, anywhere.

TM is not a lifestyle—it's a technique. You don't have to change your lifestyle in order to learn TM. Just learn it, practice it, and enjoy the benefits.

Comments on the TM Technique

"For me, personally, TM is like taking a vacation twice a day. After a long day at the office or teaching at the university, I feel completely refreshed and revitalized after TM."

Margaret Mitchell, M.D.
Specialist in Geriatrics
Buffalo

"TM is not only revitalizing, but it also gets you to a place where the mind thinks more comprehensively—it opens the doors to creativity. The result is that you find yourself taking bold new steps in directions you might not have taken before."

Stanley J. Goodman
CEO (ret.), The May Department Stores Co.
President, Top Management Services
St. Louis

"I started TM to help my career and there has been no question that it has done just that. I'm better able to handle pressure and I'm more clear and creative. But over the years the greatest benefit has been to my family life—which has become very rich and full."

Donald Weber
Chairman and President
Financial Guardian, Inc.
Kansas City

"I find that the two 20-minute periods of TM give me an inner calm, great energy, and far more presence of mind with which to serve the people of God. TM involves no faith or belief and may be practiced with confidence by any religious person."

Father Kevin Joyce
Faculty of St. Joseph's College Seminary
Mountain View, California;
Director of the Permanent Deaconate
Diocese of San Jose

"I find that I get more done since learning TM. My energy is less scattered and I can focus on things more quickly. Also my health has improved. As a school teacher and an administrator for over 30 years, I recommend TM highly to anyone."

Dr. Norman Brust
Superintendent, Afton School District
St. Louis

"I had a terrible problem with anger. I would be quick to snap and I was always tense. After I started TM, I began thinking more clearly before I would act. The anger started to decrease and I felt more peace and happiness at home."

Conley Smith, 17
The St. Paul School
Covington, Louisiana

Chapter 2
Unfolding
Full Mental Potential—
And Using It

TM is not just a technique to reduce stress. It is much more than that. TM is a practical procedure for unfolding full mental potential—and using it.

We are practical people. We have to be. Every day there are pressures, deadlines, and commitments to meet.

There's a business deal to close, children to send off to school, an exam to prepare for. And there are big plans for the future.

So is it practical to take time to consider developing mental potential—much less act on it—when there's so much to accomplish with so little time?

Perhaps intuitively we've always known that we weren't using our full potential in life, but due to the immediate demands on our time and energy, we've had to put these considerations off to a distant future.

This is being practical, is it not?

Hardly.

If There's a Choice

Psychologists and psychiatrists estimate that we use between five and ten percent of our mental potential. And there are days when even that figure may seem a bit generous.

If you had a choice, wouldn't you prefer drawing upon more of your creativity and intelligence to solve a problem at work; or organize a household; or take an exam at school?

What could be more practical than having a clear, organized mind; or the ability to learn rapidly and remember things accurately; or the capacity for broad comprehension along with the ability to focus sharply for long periods of time?

Nothing could be more practical, and therefore nothing is more practical than developing full mental potential—and using it.

How do we unfold full mental potential through TM?

Quite naturally. We simply gain access to the reservoir of energy, creativity, and intelligence that is located deep within everyone at the source of thought. To understand how this is possible, first we'll start with a few common experiences.

Excited Mind/Settled Mind

Two executives are examining the final draft of a business transaction over lunch at a crowded restaurant.

A student is working on a math problem in front of the television set.

Neither the executives nor the student are

meeting with much success. Why? Too much noise. Where there is more noise, there is more confusion. Where there is greater silence, there is more orderliness, more intelligence.

So, the executives meet later in a quiet conference room to complete the details and the student goes to his room to study.

Whenever we have something important to do, like balance a checkbook or study for a class; or whenever we have something important to say, like a heart-to-heart talk with a son or daughter, we always find a quiet environment which is conducive to the mind becoming settled. Because when the mind is allowed to settle down, it naturally grows in clarity, comprehension, and decisiveness.

What Is the Purpose of TM?

Just this: Due to the busy pace of daily life, it's often not possible to get away to a quiet environment. And even if we are able to, then because of the build-up of stress and tension, the mind still doesn't settle down naturally.

What is needed is a way to develop the ability for the mind to remain clear and settled and use its full potential at all times—even in the midst of the most hectic activity.

That's the purpose of TM. It's a simple technique that allows the active mind to settle down—and continue settling down—until it reaches its own perfectly calm, collected, self-referral state, where the body is deeply rested and the mind is silent, unbounded, and fully awake.

Moreover, it's practical. The TM technique can be practiced anywhere, at anytime. Whether it's been a hectic work day or a relaxing Sunday, whether you're just home from an all-day business meeting or a weekend fishing trip, you can practice TM and benefit from this settled state of awareness.

And what exactly is this most settled state?

It is the state of the full potential of consciousness—a silent reservoir of unlimited creativity and intelligence found deep within the mind. And this reservoir, as we'll see later, is the same as the source of unlimited creativity and intelligence found deep within nature itself.

"Optimum Level of Mental Competence"

Dr. Christopher J. Hegarty is a nationally-renowned management consultant. He is the featured speaker at over 90 business conferences a year on developing the fundamentals of competence. His client list includes the chief executives at IBM, AT&T, Blue Cross, Xerox, and the United Airlines Pilots Association. He has also been practicing the TM technique for 12 years.

Dr. Hegarty tells his audiences:

"The world is changing so fast, with so much new information to process, that to survive in business today—much less succeed—demands the use of your full mental potential.

"I consider the TM program to be the single most effective technique available for developing this optimum level of mental competence.

"This is because TM removes the stress and 'debris' from your mind and nervous system. And it gives you access to your own deepest resources—what I have found to be an unlimited reservoir of inner energy and creative intelligence."

Thought Is the Basis of Activity...

What—and where—is this reservoir that Dr. Hegarty and millions of other individuals experience twice daily through TM?

Let's analyze it step by step.

Thought is the basis of activity. For example, the design of a home begins with the thoughts of an architect. A legal brief begins with the thoughts of an attorney. An organized household is based on the thoughts of the parents.

The clearer, more creative, and more intelligent the thought, the more successful is the architectural design, the legal brief, the family's day.

What can make thought more intelligent and more powerful?

As Maharishi Mahesh Yogi, the founder of the Transcendental Meditation program, explains, contact with the inner reservoir of energy and intelligence, contact with the source of thought.

Thought: Energy and Intelligence

All day, every day we think innumerable thoughts. From the moment we wake up in the morning to the time we sleep at night, the mind is constantly thinking thoughts:

"Time to get the kids off to school."
"Who won the game last night?"
"Sandra Wright called for the data file."

Now, is there anything common to these thoughts—and all the different thoughts that we think?

Yes. *Energy* and *intelligence*.

• Energy—because all thoughts move; one thought follows another. This movement implies energy.

• Intelligence—because the energy takes a particular direction.

This means that all thoughts express some degree of energy and intelligence. And all day, every day, we are constantly thinking thoughts. That means we are constantly generating impulses of energy and intelligence.

What is the source of all this energy and intelligence? From where do thoughts arise?

While it is true that the stimulus for a particular thought may be a book or a conversation or a movie, the fact is, thoughts—energy and intelligence—arise from somewhere within us, from somewhere deep within the mind.

Where?

Source of Thought

As we discussed earlier the mind can be:
  • very noisy and excited;
  • quiet and settled; or
  • perfectly settled and silent.

As the mind settles down it naturally increases in creativity, intelligence, and power. The deepest level of the mind is the field of maximum energy and intelligence.

It is here that we locate an unbounded reservoir of pure energy, and creative intelligence. It is from here that all thoughts arise. This is the source of thought.

Maharishi explains that the source of thought is the field of pure consciousness, a self-referral level of awareness where consciousness is open only to itelf—awake to its own full potential. It is silent, yet ready to function with maximum dynamism, clarity, and orderliness.

TM is a simple, natural procedure—requiring neither concentration nor control—for refining mental activity and directly experiencing the source of thought.

TM and Science

What does science tell us about TM? From physiology, biology, and chemistry we learn that TM dissolves stress and promotes health and longevity. From psychology we learn that memory improves, learning ability increases, and intelligence grows.

And from both modern physics and TM we learn something else: We learn of the deep connection between man and nature.

We learn that the source of intelligence within man is the same as the source of the intelligence within nature. And that man has access to the unlimited creativity and intelligence of nature in his own life. We learn what it means to unfold full mental potential—and use it.

To understand this connection between man and nature, we first need a little background in physics.

Modern Physics Discovers the Unified Field (And What It Means to You)

Physics investigates nature. Man is a part of nature. So what can physics tell us about nature that can help us understand the potential of man?

First we'll review recent developments in physics and then relate them to ourselves.

Observe nature—a maple tree or a galaxy of stars or an atom—and you observe the display of nature's intelligence. Everywhere in nature we see perfect orderliness, unfathomable energy, unlimited creativity, infinite organizing power.

What is its source? Physics tells us that nature is structured in layers; that within the molecules are atoms, and within atoms are subatomic particles. The deeper the layer, the greater the energy and organizing power.

The quest of science has always been to uncover deeper levels of nature's functioning, and ultimately to discover the source of the tree, the galaxy, the atom—the very source of the universe.

Four Fundamental Forces of Nature

Thirty years ago the basis of the universe was

seen to be the four fundamental forces in nature and the so-called "matter fields."

They constituted everything in the universe. (Note: The four forces are: Electromagnetism, which accounts for such things as electricity and chemical reactions; the weak force, which is responsible for such phenomena as radioactive decay; the strong force, which holds the nucleus of an atom together; and gravity, which keeps objects earthbound and planets in orbit.)

Recently, physicists have uncovered even more powerful, more unified levels of nature, such as the "electro-weak unification," at the basis of these four forces.

Discovery of the Source: the Unified Field

And now the source of all the force and matter fields in the universe has been glimpsed by modern science in the supersymmetric unified field theories of physics.

It is called the unified field of natural law. It is a field of pure energy and intelligence which underlies everything in creation and which is responsible for all forms and phenomena in the universe.

According to physics, the entire universe emerges from the "self-interacting dynamics" of the unified field. And it is from the unified field that the entire universe is governed.

Difficult to picture? Here's an analogy: The unified field is like the sap within a tree. The sap, while colorless, odorless, and formless itself, is nonetheless the source of the fragrant, red flower; the shiny, green leaf; the leathery, brown stem.

The sap permeates the entire tree, manifesting itself as flower, leaf, and stem. In the same way, the unified field underlies and pervades the universe. It is the source of the infinite energy, creativity, and intelligence displayed in nature. It is the source of everything in the universe, including man.

Now what does this mean to you?

The Field of Intelligence Connecting Man and Nature

The unified field deep within nature is a field of unlimited energy, creativity, and intelligence. The source of thought deep within the individual is also a field of unlimited energy, creativity, and intelligence.

Is there a connection between them? Yes.

Maharishi: "Modern physics has recently glimpsed the unified field of all the laws of nature.

"Since ancient times the unified field has been described by Vedic Science, a complete science of consciousness, as the field of pure consciousness, the field of infinite energy, creativity, and intelligence underlying man and nature. Through TM, pure consciousness—the unified field—can be enlivened at the source of thought deep within the mind of every human being.

"This means that man can display the infinite creativity, intelligence, and dynamism of nature in his own life. This is his natural birthright."

Quantum Physics and Consciousness

Dr. John S. Hagelin, a member of an elite group of scientists who are at the forefront of research in the unified field, agrees.

Dr. Hagelin is an expert on supersymmetric unified quantum field theories and has published over 40 papers on unified field theories in leading physics journals. He received his doctorate in physics from Harvard, and has conducted research at two of the leading laboratories in the world for advanced particle physics—the European Laboratory for Particle Physics (CERN) in Geneva, Switzerland, and the Stanford Linear Accelerator Center in Palo Alto, California.

Since 1976, Dr. Hagelin has also studied Maharishi's descriptions of pure consciousness—the source of thought—in the light of modern physics.

Recent advances in quantum physics, Dr. Hagelin says, provide "substantial evidence that the unified field and pure consciousness are not two separate fields, but one and the same." As chairman of the department of physics and director of the doctoral program in physics at Maharishi International University in Fairfield, Iowa, Dr. Hagelin is a recognized world authority on unified field theories and a pre-eminent scholar in the dynamics of human consciousness.

Origin in the Unified Field

Dr. Hagelin: "It is clear that the unified field is

ultimately the origin of all attributes in the universe. Any property of existence—electric charge or color charge—must have its dynamical origin in the structure of the unified field itself.

"The properties of intelligence, dynamism, and self-interaction can also be located in the structure of the unified field, suggesting a link between the unified field and the 'ground state' or most fundamental state of consciousness.

"When one examines the properties of the unified field in detail, one discovers all the properties of pure consciousness."

What Does All of This Mean?

It means, as Maharishi has said, that the full potential of the human mind is the same as the total potential of nature's intelligence.

It means that we have the innate capacity to utilize and display the unlimited energy, creativity, and intelligence of nature in our own life.

And for this we only need to restore the natural connection—through the practice of TM—between the active thinking mind and the source of thought; between the active mind and the unified field.

When we make that connection we develop creativity and intelligence, reduce stress and fatigue, and enjoy greater progress and achievement in life. We gain the support of nature in everything we do.

And this is why TM is called the Maharishi Technology of the Unified Field.

Self-Referral State of Awareness

Maharishi comments: "In Transcendental Meditation, the conscious mind comes to a state of self-referral awareness, which is the simplest form of human awareness where consciousness is open only to itself. This self-referral state of consciousness is the unified field of natural law.

"The supersymmetric unified field theories of physics have glimpsed this state of unity, which, through its own self-interacting dynamics, expresses itself as diversified forms and phenomena in creation.

"When the conscious mind identifies itself with the unified field through the process of Transcendental Meditation, then human awareness is open to its own full potential, which is the total potential of nature's intelligence.

"As a result, thinking and action spontaneously become more and more in accord with the evolutionary power of natural law. By enlivening this most basic level, Transcendental Meditation is that one simple procedure which can raise the life of every individual to its full dignity in which perfect health, happiness, and success are the natural features of daily life."

THEORY

Knowledge of the Unified Field as the Self-Interacting Level of Nature's Functioning

QUANTUM PHYSICS

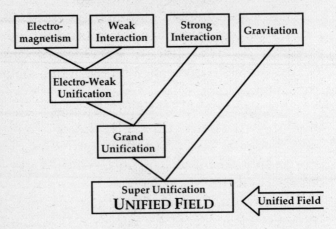

Progress in theoretical physics during the past decade has led to a progressively more unified understanding of the fundamental forces of nature. This has culminated in the recent discovery of completely unified field theories.

PRACTICE

Experience of the Unified Field in the
Self-Referral State of Consciousness through
Transcendental Meditation

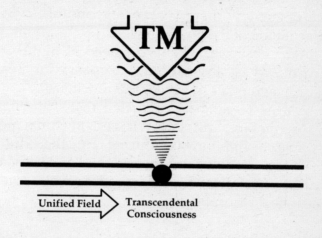

Transcendental Meditation allows the active
thinking mind to settled down to transcendental
consciousness, the field of pure intelligence, where
the mind is silent, unbounded, and fully awake
within itself. This self-referral state of consciousness
is the unified field of natural law.

Science Studies TM:
Mind/Body Connection

When scientists decided to research the effects of TM, they looked to the body.

Why?

Because of the intimate connection between mind and body. They knew that for every state of consciousness there is a corresponding style of functioning of the physiology.

(For example, when you sleep at night your brain waves slow down, as does your heart, breath, and other physiological functions.)

So the researchers predicted that if the mind does, in fact, quiet down and become more expanded, more awake during TM, then due to the close coordination between mind and body, the entire physiology must change as well. And it must be measurable.

The First Research on TM

The first scientist to study the physiological effects of TM was Dr. Robert Keith Wallace at UCLA in 1968.

Dr. Wallace found that during TM the entire system gained a unique and profound state of rest and relaxation. He further observed biochemical changes indicative of reduced stress and changes in EEG, or brain wave patterns, which indicated a state of "heightened inner wakefulness," or restful alertness.

A State of Restful Alertness

Analyzing his data and comparing it to research on the three major states of consciousness, Dr. Wallace arrived at this conclusion:

The TM technique produces a fourth major state of consciousness, a unique state of "restful alertness" different from waking, dreaming, and sleeping states of consciousness, but natural and vital to the health and well-being of the individual.

Dr. Wallace's findings were published in the March 1970 issue of *Science*.

Since that initial study there have been over 350 scientific research studies on TM, conducted at 160 independent universities and research institutions, such as Harvard Medical School, Stanford Medical School, and UCLA.

Much of the research has been published in leading scientific journals, including *Science*, *The American Journal of Physiology*, *The International Journal of Neuroscience*, and *Psychosomatic Medicine*.

The research has documented the effects of the TM program in every area of life, including mind, body, behavior, and society.

Brain Wave Coherence

One of the most significant findings has been the discovery that TM produces a unique ordering or coherence in brain wave patterns between the different parts of the brain. And the longer a person practices TM, the higher the EEG coherence.

Dr. Wallace, who today is one of the world's leading authorities on the scientific research on the TM program, explained the meaning of this finding:

"The higher EEG coherence produced during TM indicates that the technique 'optimizes brain functioning.' This means that the brain functions in a more coherent, integrated style during TM than during the usual waking, dreaming, and sleeping states of consciousness.

"Many psychological studies have shown that, among other findings, this higher EEG coherence gained during TM is associated with increased intelligence, increased creativity, and higher moral reasoning."

What is the cause of the EEG coherence?

Dr. Wallace: "The increased orderliness and integration between the different parts of the brain corresponds to the direct experience of the self-referral state of pure consciousness—the unified field—gained during TM."

Using Full Mental Potential

For the scientist, increased brain wave coherence means "optimizing brain functioning."

For the TM practitioner, increased brain wave coherence means developing—and using—full mental potential. And using full mental potential means enjoying the state of enlightenment in daily life.

The following five research charts are a few of the many scientific studies conducted on the benefits of the TM technique for developing mental potential. The charts represent the average benefits of the group studied.

GREATER ORDERLINESS OF BRAIN FUNCTIONING
INCREASED EEG COHERENCE

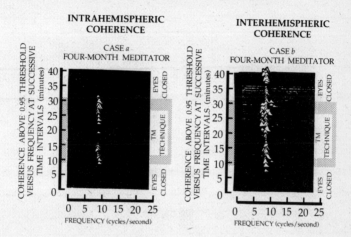

INTRAHEMISPHERIC COHERENCE

CASE *a*
FOUR-MONTH MEDITATOR

INTERHEMISPHERIC COHERENCE

CASE *b*
FOUR-MONTH MEDITATOR

Higher levels of EEG coherence have been positively correlated with physiological, psychological, and emotional factors that indicate optimization of brain functioning. The results show that EEG coherence—a quantitative index of long range spatial ordering of the brain waves—increases between and within the cerebral hemispheres during the Transcendental Meditation technique.

P.H. Levine, "The Coherence Spectral Array (COSPAR) and Its Application to the Study of Spatial Ordering in the EEG," *Proceedings of the San Diego Biomedical Symposium*, vol. 15 (USA: 1976).

BROADER COMPREHENSION
AND IMPROVED ABILITY TO FOCUS
INCREASED FIELD INDEPENDENCE

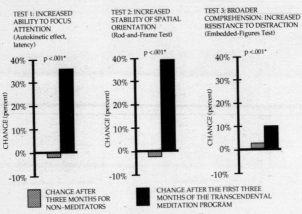

TEST 1: INCREASED ABILITY TO FOCUS ATTENTION (Autokinetic effect, latency)

TEST 2: INCREASED STABILITY OF SPATIAL ORIENTATION (Rod-and-Frame Test)

TEST 3: BROADER COMPREHENSION: INCREASED RESISTANCE TO DISTRACTION (Embedded-Figures Test)

CHANGE AFTER THREE MONTHS FOR NON–MEDITATORS

CHANGE AFTER THE FIRST THREE MONTHS OF THE TRANSCENDENTAL MEDITATION PROGRAM

*Analysis of variance-meditation effect.

Field independence has been associated with a greater ability to assimilate and structure experience, greater organization of mind and cognitive clarity, improved memory, greater creative expression, and a stable internal frame of reference. The results show that practice of the TM technique develops greater field independence. This improvement in TM meditators is remarkable because it was previously thought that these basic perceptual abilities do not improve beyond early adulthood.

Reference I: K.R. Pelletier, "Influence of Transcendental Meditation upon Autokinetic Perception," *Perceptual Motor Skills* 39 (U.S.A.: 1974): 1031-1034. Reference II: M.C. Dillbeck, Assimakis, et al., "Longitudinal Effects of the Transcendental Meditation and TM-Sidhi Program on Cognitive Ability and Cognitive Style," *Perceptual and Motor Skills* 62 (U.S.A.: 1986): 731-738.

INCREASED MENTAL POTENTIAL IN ADULTS

INCREASED INTELLIGENCE

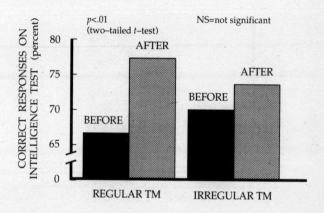

Several studies have indicated that intelligence increases over time as a result of participation in the TM program. This is noteworthy because fluid intelligence, which is generally measured by nonverbal intelligence tests such as the one used in this study, usually does not improve after adolescence and often declines after the age of 20 years. The study shown above followed TM meditators for 16 months after they received instruction in the TM technique. Regularity of TM practice was found to correlate significantly with changes in intelligence score.

A.S. Tjoa, "Meditation, Neuroticism and Intelligence: A Follow Up," *Gedrag, Tijdschrift voor Psychologie* 3 (The Netherlands: 1975): 167-182.

IMPROVED ACADEMIC PERFORMANCE IN GRADUATE STUDENTS

IMPROVED EXAM SCORES

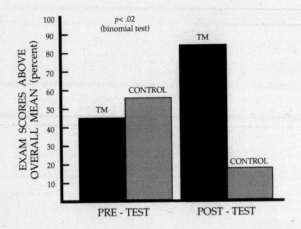

Using a random assignment design, this study found that graduate students practicing the TM technique regularly for six months scored significantly higher on academic examinations than control students in comparison to previous performance. These findings extend previous work that showed similar effects at the high school and undergraduate levels.

P. Kember, "The Transcendental Meditation Technique and Postgraduate Performance," *British Journal of Educational Psychology* 55 (England: 1985): 164-166.

INCREASED MENTAL POTENTIAL IN UNIVERSITY STUDENTS

INCREASED LEARNING ABILITY

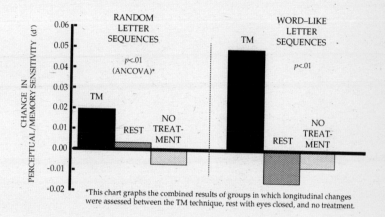

*This chart graphs the combined results of groups in which longitudinal changes were assessed between the TM technique, rest with eyes closed, and no treatment.

These results indicate that the TM practice directly improves the ability to learn. This finding is particularly significant in view of the common belief among psychologists that basic learning ability cannot be improved beyond late adolescence.

Michael Dillbeck, "Meditation and Flexibility of Visual Perception and Verbal Problem Solving," *Memory and Cognition* 10 (U.S.A.: 1982): 207-215.

CHAPTER 3

Healthy Mind/ Healthy Body

"It is fortunate for the field of health that one technique exists to take care of the very basis of an individual's life—pure consciousness—and thereby to restore and maintain perfect health on all levels of mind, body, and surroundings."

—Maharishi

Over 380 billion dollars is spent on health care in the United States each year—nearly 10 percent of the entire gross national product (GNP) for the country. That means one dollar of every ten earned in America is spent on health care. And the amount continues to escalate.

What is the money used for? Preventing illnesses? Promoting the health and well-being of Americans, one of the wealthiest and most creative people in the world?

Unfortunately, no. It is used primarily for treating diseases. And according to many health experts, nine out of ten of these diseases could have been prevented.

How?

Essentially, by preventing stress-based diseases, which account for the vast majority of all of the maladies of mankind, including nuisance illnesses such as the common cold and serious disorders such as heart disease and many forms of cancer.

What Causes Stress?

Stress is not a deadline to meet at work, a crying baby, a law school entrance exam. Stress is how we react, physically and mentally, to those pressures.

Some days we're better at it, some days we're not. If we've slept well at night and awaken fresh and rested, we're apt to handle any demand during the day far better than if we run into it, headlong, on a Friday afternoon at the end of a long and tiring week.

Stress can be understood as any structural or material abnormality in the body (tight neck muscles, high blood pressure, tension headaches, etc.) that is caused by overloading the machinery of experience, the senses.

Any overload can cause it. The flash of a bulb from a camera can create some stress in the eyes. Too much excitement can cause stress—or not enough rest. Any experience, positive or negative, can create stress if the system is unable to handle it.

"But Stress Is the Spice of Life..."

"But stress is the spice of life," you say. "People who enjoy the continual stimulation of new challenges, new responsibilities, new pressures would hate to live without stress."

It is true that new challenges are essential to a creative, dynamic person. Eliminating stress from life does not mean eliminating challenges.

It means, rather, eliminating the negative effect of these challenges, e.g., fatigue, tension, headaches, indigestion, insomnia, which restrict our capacity to enjoy life.

How to Manage Stress?

How, then, can we advance our career and fulfill our family commitments without becoming victims of stress?

There are many "stress management techniques" available today which try to minimize stress by training executives, housewives, or students how to better organize their responsibilities and environment.

These techniques advise how to avoid high pressure situations, recommend mental imagery exercises, and advocate changes in lifestyle—such as exercise and diet—to reduce stress. Some even suggest de-escalating career goals.

Are these the basics of stress management?

No.

They are helpful in their own right, but they are not the "bottom line" on stress management.

What is the bottom line?

The deep rest gained during TM.

Twenty minutes of TM provides a unique and profound state of rest and relaxation. This rest, gained on a twice daily basis, allows the body to throw off stress and fatigue that has built up over years. It helps to normalize high blood pressure, provide relief from insomnia, reduce high cholesterol levels, improve bronchial asthma, increase reaction time—even improve athletic performance. The deep rest gained during TM allows the body to rejuvenate itself.

Without this deep rest, we can only hope to "manage" stress and work to organize our life to cope with the problems of modern living, not solve them.

Don't Manage Stress, *Eliminate* It

With this rest, we don't just "manage" stress, we eliminate it. We promote health and vitality, clarity of mind and orderliness of thinking. Then we are better equipped to meet all of our responsibilities and commitments in life, not reduce them. And we grow in the capacity to enjoy life to its fullest.

These are the benefits of TM for eliminating stress. We know stress contributes to aging. What, then, are the effects of TM on aging?

TM Over Time: Younger Biological Age

Dr. Ronald Jevning is associate professor of medicine at the University of California at Irvine. Since 1973, Dr. Jevning has studied the biochemical effects of TM on stress and aging. He has published over 40 research papers in leading scientific journals and his research has been supported by grants from the National Institutes of Health and the American Heart Association.

Dr. Jevning says:

"I am often asked about the benefits of the TM technique and if there is any difference between TM and ordinary rest or so-called 'relaxation techniques.'

"The answer is, 'Yes, absolutely.'

"There are many studies that have clearly distinguished the effects of TM from ordinary rest or relaxation. The research has shown that if someone tells you to simply 'relax' or 'rest,' very little happens.

"Research on TM, on the other hand, has shown the technique to be a highly effective means to gain a very deep state of rest at will which is useful for enhancing mental and physical health.

"But the most exciting new development has been studies on the long-term practice of TM. This research shows that the practice of TM over time can actually promote a younger biological age."

The Aging Process

To understand how TM could promote a younger biological age first requires an understanding of the aging process itself:

Bill is 48 years old according to his birth certificate, but his doctor knows otherwise. His doctor knows that because of stress at work Bill has the physiology of a 60-year-old. The doctor recommends that Bill reduce his workload, stop smoking, and take special medication for his blood pressure.

John, on the other hand, is 49 years old and in good shape. His doctor says that John has the physiology of a man five years younger. He gets a clean bill of health.

There is a difference between chronological age and biological age. Chronological age is the number of years an individual has lived; biological age is an indication of his overall state of health as compared to population norms.

Scientists use a battery of tests, such as measurements of systolic blood pressure, auditory threshold, and near-point vision, to distinguish a person's biological age from his actual chronological age. This is because people age at different rates.

According to most theories, the causes of biological aging are complex. They include heredity, the stress of modern living, and prior illnesses. But it all adds up to wear and tear on the system.

Research on TM and Aging

Scientists have long-recognized TM as highly effective in reducing wear and tear and stress on a day-to-day basis. In recent years they have become very interested in determining what cumulative effects the long-term practice of the TM technique has on an individual's health and biological age.

The first scientist to study the effects of TM on aging was Dr. Robert Keith Wallace, the same physiologist who pioneered TM research as a graduate student at UCLA in 1968.

Twelve years after his first TM study was published in *Science*, Dr. Wallace published his breakthrough research on TM and aging in the *International Journal of Neuroscience* (1982).

12 Years Younger...

Dr. Wallace found that subjects with an average chronological age of 50 years old who had been practicing TM for over five years had a biological age 12 years younger than their chronological age. They had the physiology of an average 38-year-old.

Several of the subjects in the study were found to have a biological age 27 years younger than their chronological age. (This study has since been replicated several times.)

Is this surprising?

Dr. Wallace: "It's not surprising when you consider that all the major factors associated with longevity have been shown to improve with the regular practice of the TM technique.

"TM has been shown to significantly improve cardiovascular health, work satisfaction, positive health habits, physical function, happiness rating, self-health rating, intelligence, and mental health.

"The result is a younger biological age."

The Bottom Line on TM and Health

What is the practical advantage of a younger biological age? Among the many benefits: less sickness and fewer hospital admissions.

A study of a five year period (1981-1985) of data from a major insurance carrier in the United States on a group of 2000 TM practitioners found that the TM group had less than half of the hospital admissions and outpatient visits of other professional groups.

In addition, TM practitioners over 40 years of age were found to have an even higher percentage reduction in insurance utilization than the controls for their age group.

The conclusion?

As you grow older, it's not only possible to become healthier—its even possible to grow younger biologically as well.

The following is a review of some of the scientific research conducted on physiological effects during the practice of TM and its benefits for health in daily life.

NATURAL CHANGE IN BREATHING
LOWER BREATH RATE

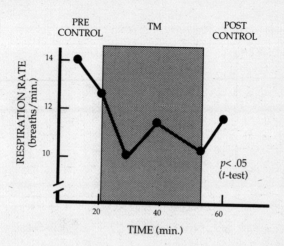

Subjects were measured for changes in breathing rate during the practice of the TM technique. Breath rate fell from about 14 breaths per minute to about 11 breaths per minute, indicating the TM technique produces a state of rest and relaxation. The change in breath rate is natural, effortless, and comfortable.

R.K. Wallace, et. al. "A Wakeful Hypometabolic Physiologic State," *American Journal of Physiology* 221 (1971): 795-799.

BIOCHEMISTRY OF DEEP REST
REDUCED CORTISOL

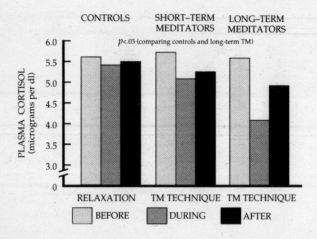

Plasma cortisol is a stress hormone. The result of the study shows that plasma cortisol decreased during the TM technique, whereas it did not change significantly in control subjects during ordinary relaxation.

R. Jevning, A.F. Wilson, and J.M. Davidson, "Adrenocortical Activity During Meditation," *Hormones and Behavior* 10, no. 1 (U.S.A.: 1978) 54-60.

PHYSIOLOGY OF DEEP REST

PHYSIOLOGICAL CHANGES
DURING THE TM TECHNIQUE

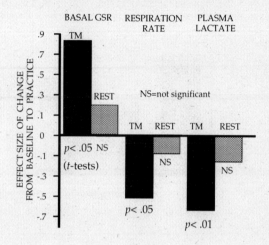

A meta-analysis of all available research studies on the TM technique found that during the practice, TM meditators display a deeper state of relaxation than control subjects during eyes-closed rest as measured by basal skin resistance, respiration rates, and plasma lactate levels.

M. C. Dillbeck and D.W. Orme-Johnson, "Physiological Differences Between Transcendental Meditation and Rest," *American Psychologist,* (USA) in press.

BENEFICIAL EFFECTS
ON BRONCHIAL ASTHMA

IMPROVED ABILITY TO BREATHE
AND REDUCED SYMPTOMS OF ASTHMA

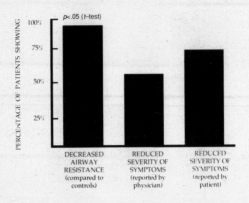

Bronchial asthma is one of a group of diseases the severity of which has been consistently correlated with the level of psychological stress of the individual. The results show that the TM technique is beneficial for patients with bronchial asthma, indicating its effectiveness in reducing stress.

Reference I: R. Honsberger and A.F. Wilson, "The Effect of Transcendental Meditation upon Bronchial Asthma," *Clinical Research* 22, no. 2 (U.S.A.: 1973). Reference II: R. Honsberger and A.F. Wilson, "Transcendental Meditation in Treating Asthma," *Respiratory Therapy: The Journal of Inhalation Technology* 3, no. 6 (U.S.A.: 1973): 79-80. Reference III: A.F. Wilson, R. Honsberger, J.T. Chiu, and H.S. Novey, "Transcendental Meditation and Asthma," *Respiration* 32 (U.S.A.: 1973): 74-80.

IMPROVED CARDIOVASCULAR HEALTH

LOWER SYSTOLIC BLOOD PRESSURE

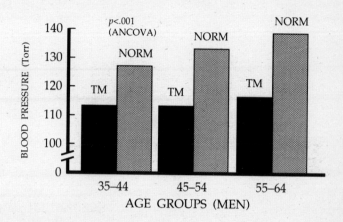

Systolic blood pressure, the pressure in the blood vessels at the end of a heart beat, was measured in 112 TM meditators and compared to known values for the general population. The results showed the TM meditators had significantly lower blood pressures than the general population. Furthermore, the long-term meditators had lower blood pressures than the short-term meditators in this study.

R.K. Wallace, J. Sliver, P. Mills, M. Dillbeck, and D. Wagoner, "Systolic Blood Pressure and Long-Term Practice of the Transcendental Meditation and TM-Sidhi Program: Effects of TM on Systolic Blood Pressure," *Psychosomatic Medicine* 45, no. 1 (U.S.A.: 1983): 41-46.

REDUCED CARDIOVASCULAR RISK FACTOR

REDUCED CHOLESTEROL LEVELS

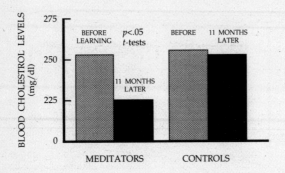

Stress and anxiety are among the factors that can increase cholesterol levels. This study tested subjects with high blood cholesterol levels at the beginning of the experiment and 11 months later. The subjects who practiced the TM technique showed a significant drop in the level of cholesterol in their blood, while the control group showed very little decrease. Diet was controlled in this study.

Reference I: M. J. Cooper and M. M. Aygen, "Transcendental Meditation in the Management of Hypercholesterolemia," *Journal of Human Stress* 5, 4 (1979): 24-27. Reference II: M. J. Cooper and M. M. Aygen, "Effect of Transcendental Meditation on Serum Cholesterol and Blood Pressure," *Harefuah, the Journal of the Israel Medical Association,* 95, 1 (1978): 1-2.

BENEFICIAL EFFECTS ON THE AGING PROCESS
YOUNGER BIOLOGICAL AGE

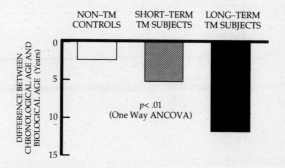

The Adult Growth Examination is a standard test for biological age. It was given to 73 TM meditators and 11 non-meditating controls. The results showed the long-term meditators to be 12 years younger than their chronological age, the short-term TM meditators were five years younger than their chronological age, while the controls were 2.2 years younger. The study was statistically controlled for diet and exercise.

R.K. Wallace, M. Dillbeck, E. Jacobe, and B. Harrington, "The Effects of the Transcendental Meditation and TM-Sidhi Program on the Aging Process," *International Journal of Neuroscience*, 16, no. 1 (U.S.A.: 1982): 53-58.

REDUCED NEED FOR MEDICAL CARE
DECREASED DOCTOR VISITS

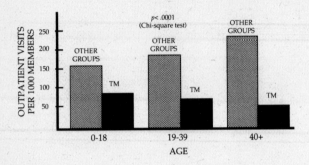

A study of health insurance statistics on over 2000 people practicing the TM program over a five-year period found that the TM meditators consistently had less than half the doctor visits than other groups of comparable age, gender, profession and insurance terms. The difference between the TM and non-TM groups increased in older age brackets.

Reference I: D.W. Orme-Johnson, "Medical Care Utilization and the Transcendental Meditation Program," *Psychosomatic Medicine*, in press. Reference II: D.W. Orme-Johnson and R. Schneider, "Reduced Health Care Utilization in Transcendental Meditation Practitioners," presented at the conference of the Society for Behavioral Medicine, Washington, D.C., March 22, 1987.

REDUCED NEED FOR MEDICAL CARE
DECREASED HOSPITALIZATION

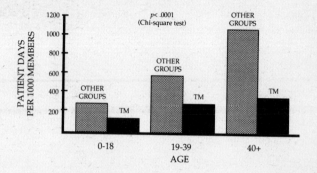

A study of health insurance statistics on over 2000 peo-ple practicing the TM program over a five-year period found that the TM meditators consistently had less than half the hospitalization than other groups of comparable age, gender, profession and insurance terms. The differ-ence between the TM and non-TM groups increased in older age brackets. In addition, the TM meditators had fewer incidents of illness in 17 medical treatment cate-gories, including 87 percent less hospitalization for heart disease and 55 percent less for cancer.

Reference I: D.W. Orme-Johnson, "Medical Care Utilization and the Transcendental Meditation Program," *Psychosomatic Medicine,* in press. Reference II: D.W. Orme-Johnson and R. Schneider, "Reduced Health Care Utilization in Transcendental Meditation Practitioners," presented at the conference of the Society for Behavioral Medicine, Washington, D.C., March 22, 1987.

CHAPTER 4

Ideal Relationships

I t's almost 6:00 p.m. and Barry Pitt has put in a full day at work. As vice-president of a large retail business in Redford, a suburb of Detroit, Barry oversees more than 100 employees, and spends most of each day in meetings with his managers, talking on the telephone, trouble-shooting, and, when there's time, working the floor with the employees.

His store is open until 9:00 p.m. tonight, but Barry, who's been at work since 8:00 a.m. has finished his work for the day. As he shuts the door to his office, Barry thinks of the rush hour traffic at its peak on the Southfield Freeway. He smiles. He's not going anywhere just now.

Settling down in the chair behind his desk, loosening his tie, Barry closes his eyes and begins his afternoon TM practice. Twenty minutes later, rested and refreshed, he collects his coat and briefcase and heads home for dinner.

For Jane, Barry's wife, it seems as if she has been in the car all day: driving the kids to school, grocery shopping, taking the car to the garage to have the *muffler checked, home for a quick lunch, and then off to Oakland University where she's taking a post-graduate course in music.*

At 3:00 p.m. Jane's back home. There's house-work to do, dinner to prepare, and a paper to write for class. But the house is quiet and she has half an hour until her two children come home from school. Sitting down and making herself comfort-able on the family room sofa, she closes her eyes and begins her afternoon TM practice. Twenty min-utes later, feeling revitalized, she greets Jesse, 8, and Joanna, 5, as they burst in the front door from school.

Barry and Jane have been practicing TM twice daily for over 10 years. Barry says it has made him more efficient and productive at work. Jane says that her musical and artistic abilities have improved significantly. Both agree that it has helped make their family life far more satisfying and enjoyable.

The World Is as We Are

"A strong mind is tolerant; a weak mind is easi-ly overcome by the surroundings."

—Maharishi

It's a common experience: One morning you wake up as tired as when you went to sleep. The day moves slowly, complications arise, problems seem to be overwhelming. You feel worried; rela-tionships suffer.

But the next morning, after a deep sleep, you feel fresh and alert. The circumstances of the previous day may remain the same, but your evaluation of them differs dramatically. You are more relaxed, yet more energetic, more productive. Relationships are smoother, more harmonious.

Why the difference?

Basically, it's because the world is as you are.

Put on green glasses and everything appears green. Put on yellow glasses and everything is yellow.

Look through tired eyes with an anxious mind and your vision is clouded with problems, many of which, in reality, may not exist.

Look through fresh eyes with an alert, creative mind and you are better able to see the solutions to problems that do exist. When you are fresh you possess the energy and intelligence to solve problems, and make rapid improvements in all areas of life.

What's needed?

Less stress, more energy, a clearer mind, and a fully expanded consciousness—all of which are the basis of the complete development of the mind, personality, and behavior.

Good Social Behavior

In his book, *Science of Being and Art of Living*, Maharishi writes, "Really good social behavior between people will only be possible when their awareness is broadened, when they are able to see the whole situation, to understand each other more thoroughly, to be aware of each other's need and attempt to fulfill that need. This naturally necessitates a fully developed consciousness, a right sense of judgement, and all the qualities that only a strong and clear mind possesses."

And without this developed consciousness?

Maharishi: "Small minds always fail to perceive the whole situation and in their narrow vision create imaginary obstacles and restrictions that are neither useful to themselves nor to anyone else. Then their behavior towards others only results in misunderstanding and increase of tension."

Relationships Thrive on Giving

It's also a common experience that relationships thrive on giving. At home, it's a father giving time and attention to his children. At work, it's a manager giving proper guidance and attention to the sales trainees.

But we can only give from what we have. A father who returns home from work exhausted can hardly give his children the love and support they need.

Likewise, the manager who is anxious and short-tempered can hardly provide the necessary patience and insight to properly train his staff.

What is the solution?

TM and Relationships

To understand the effects of TM on improving personal relationships and increasing the capacity to give is just a matter of common sense.

Since we are able to think more clearly with TM, then we are in a better position to properly evaluate situations and circumstances as they arise. With a broader vision, we are naturally more tolerant and understanding.

Similarly, because we have an effective technique to eliminate stress, then we won't have to suffer from the increasing build-up of tension and fatigue. There will be less anxiety and more energy available throughout the day. And with less stress we can be more appreciative of our family, friends, and associates.

The result? Relationships naturally improve, and life becomes more enjoyable—and fulfilling.

Here's a case in point:

Tom and Sandy Kelly are the owners of Kelly and Company, a Midwest real estate and land development firm headquartered in Iowa.

Sandy recalls her experiences:

"I used to come home from work feeling absolutely exhausted. I had no energy for my family, no time for myself. My home life suffered and my business was adversely affected from too much stress and too much worry.

"I learned TM at the recommendation of an

associate. The first thing I noticed was that I had more energy during the day and that I slept better at night.

"But more than that, my relationships at home and at work improved dramatically. I found that I no longer carried the stress of the day home with me. And I was more aware of the needs of my family, as well as my clients. I now find that I am able to fulfill my commitments at home and at work without causing stress to my health or a strain in my life."

Tom adds:

"To be successful in business—and stay there—requires a tremendous amount of energy and focus. But I've always wanted my life to be more than just business at the office. When I come home after work, I want to be able to relax, spend time with my family, and really enjoy my life.

"TM develops these abilities simultaneously. I now have more energy and drive than ever before, and I am far more successful in my business. And yet, at the same time, I can leave my work at the office when I go home. I am able to take it easy and really enjoy my family."

Collective Effects

When every member of a family practices TM, the result is obvious: The quality of life improves for the whole family.

A similar influence has been found in business.

Research on companies where TM has been offered to employees on a company-wide basis has shown that productivity increases, job performance improves, there are fewer health care costs, and relationships among all the employees improve.

The following is a review of some of the research on the effects of TM for improving self-esteem, personal relationships, and corporate success.

INCREASED PRODUCTIVITY

INCREASED JOB SATISFACTION, INCREASED JOB PERFORMANCE, DECREASED DESIRE TO CHANGE JOBS

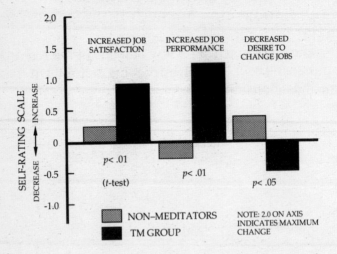

In this study subjects practicing the TM program showed significant improvements at work compared with members of a control group. Job performance and job satisfaction increased, while desire to change jobs decreased. People at every level of the organization benefited from practicing the TM program.

D.R. Frew, "Transcendental Meditation and Productivity," *Academy of Management Journal* 17, no. 2 (U.S.A.: 1974): 362-368.

IMPROVED RELATIONS AT WORK

IMPROVED RELATIONS WITH SUPERVISORS, IMPROVED RELATIONS WITH CO-WORKERS, DECREASED CLIMB ORIENTATION

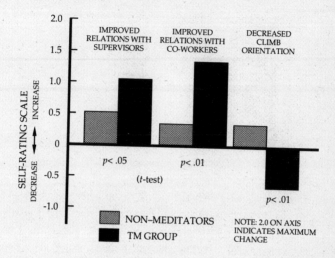

In this study subjects practicing the TM program showed significant improvements in relations with supervisors and co-workers compared with members of a control group. And while TM meditators reported that they felt less anxiety about promotion (shown by reduced climb orientation), their fellow employees saw them as moving ahead quickly. People at every level of the organization benefited from practicing TM.

D.R. Frew, "Transcendental Meditation and Productivity," *Academy of Management Journal* 17, no. 2 (U.S.A.: 1974): 362-368.

DECREASED ANXIETY
REDUCTION OF TRAIT ANXIETY

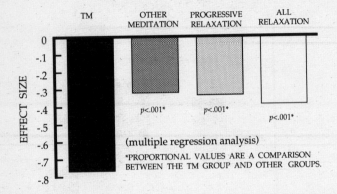

A statistical meta-analysis of all available studies—99 independent outcomes—indicated that the effect of the TM program on reducing anxiety as a character trait was approximately twice as great as that of all other meditation and relaxation techniques. Analysis also showed that the positive TM result could not be attributed to subject expectation, experimenter bias, or quality of research design.

Kenneth Eppley, Allan I. Abrams, and Jonathan Shear, "Effects of Meditation and Relaxation on Trait Anxiety: A Meta-Analysis," (Paper presented at the August 1984 Convention of the American Psychological Association, Toronto, Canada), *Scientific Research on the Transcendental Meditation and TM-Sidhi Program: Collected Papers, Vol. 4,* in press, (U.S.A.: 1985).

IMPROVED SELF CONCEPT

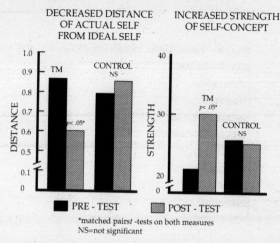

DECREASED DISTANCE OF ACTUAL SELF FROM IDEAL SELF

INCREASED STRENGTH OF SELF-CONCEPT

■ PRE - TEST   ▨ POST - TEST

*matched pairs *t* -tests on both measures
NS=not significant

One month after beginning the TM technique, subjects were found to have an improved self concept in comparison to before learning TM. As revealed by factor analysis of a role construct repertory grid, TM meditators came to experience their actual-selves as significantly closer to their ideal-selves and also developed a more strongly defined concept of their actual-selves. No similar changes were observed for matched controls.

M.J. Turnbull and H. Norris, "Effects of Transcendental Meditation on Self-Identity Indices and Personality," *British Journal of Psychology*, 73 (1982): 57-68.

DEVELOPMENT OF PERSONALITY
INCREASED SELF-ACTUALIZATION

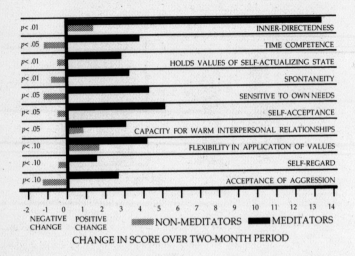

The result shows that practice of the TM technique develops self-actualization, defined in part as a high level of maturity, health, and fulfillment; a clearer perception of reality; increased integration, wholeness, and unity of person; and increased spontaneity, objectivity, and autonomy.

Reference I: Sanford Nidich, William Seeman, and Thomas Dreskin, "Influence of Transcendental Meditation: A Replication," *Journal of Counseling Psychology* 20, no. 6 (U.S.A.: 1973): 565-566. Reference II: William Seeman, Sanford Nidich, and Thomas Banta, "Influence of Transcendental Meditation on a Measure of Self-Actualization," *Journal of Counseling Psychology* 19, no. 3 (U.S.A.: 1972): 184-187.

REDUCED SUBSTANCE USAGE
REDUCED USE OF CAFFEINE, TOBACCO, ALCOHOL, MARIJUANA, AND PRESCRIBED DRUGS

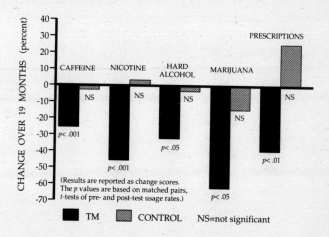

The results show the practice of the Transcendental Meditation program was associated with significant decreases in usage of a variety of active substances—prescribed and non-prescribed, addictive and non-addictive.

R. J. Monahan, "Secondary Prevention of Drug Dependence through the Transcendental Meditation Program in Metropolitan Philadelphia," *International Journal of Addictions* 12, no. 5 (U.S.A.: 1977): 729-754.

Chapter 5

Living in Accord
with Natural Law

O*ne day you are worried and tense. You feel out-of-step with the day. You miss a business connection, say the wrong thing at a meeting, you even seem to hit all the red lights when you're rushing late for an appointment.*

Another day you are feeling especially good. Everything seems to go right and click into place. You find the ideal parking place, reach the right person on the telephone, think of a perfect solution to a problem at work. The day seems to go effortlessly and enjoyably and you wonder why every day can't go at least as smoothly.

Well, why not?

Throw a tennis ball up in the air and it falls to the earth. Gravity, a law of nature.

Heat water to 212° F and it boils. A law of nature.

Water a plant, give it proper food and sunlight and it grows. Laws of nature.

The entire world, the entire universe is governed by laws of nature. Everywhere we look—at the elementary particles through an electron microscope or at the galactic life through a high-powered telescope—everything in the universe is permeated by intelligence; all activity is governed by natural law.

What is its function?

Like a strong current in a river, natural law propels life in an evolutionary direction. It is the invincible force in nature from the level of the unified field that continually creates, maintains, and evolves life.

Natural Law and You

Now, what does that have to do with you?

Everything. Because not only are electrons and galaxies subject to the laws of nature, but so is each one of us.

There are, for example, countless laws of nature which govern the functioning of your body. Align yourself with those laws—eat the right foods, exercise, and get enough rest, etc.—and your body maintains its health.

Violate those laws and you fall sick and suffer.

The key, then, to better health—actually the key to perfect health—is to attune yourself with all the laws of nature which promote growth and evolution. It's also the key to skill in action in life.

How can that be accomplished?

TM and Natural Law

It's quite easy with TM.

But before we discuss how, let's analyze the ways that you can't gain this alliance:

• By trying to intellectually understand or remember all of the different laws of nature that govern life, or

• By trying to strictly adhere to specific laws of nature.

Why? Because there are far too many laws of nature to understand, much less remember. And even if you were able to gain a little knowledge about certain laws of nature, it's no guarantee you'll be able to abide by them.

For example, there's the medical doctor, an expert in the cause of stress-related diseases, who gets sick from overwork and worry. Fully aware of the consequences of stress, nonetheless he is unable to follow his own professional advice and he overexerts.

Or the executive who is placed on a strict diet or exercise regimen by his physician for health reasons. How long does it take before he begins to compromise his routine—even though it's in his own best interest?

What is the difficulty?

To act in a completely life-supporting manner is next to impossible—unless it is natural. It can never be accomplished by trying to remember what's right, or by trying to behave in a strict, proper way.

Life in accordance with natural law must be spontaneous. And it can only be lived on the basis of a fully developed consciousness.

Living in Accord with Natural Law

TM places life in the center stream of the evolutionary power of natural law.

How?

By allowing the conscious mind to settle down to its most silent, wakeful, and fully expanded state, TM opens the awareness to the self-referral state of pure consciousness, which is the unified field of all the laws of nature.

As we discussed earlier, it is the unified field, through its "self-interacting dynamics," which expresses itself as all the diversified forms and phenomena in creation. This means that all matter, all energy, and all the laws of nature which govern all the activity in the universe spring from the unified field.

When we open our awareness to the unified field during TM, we draw upon the unlimited potential of nature at its source. The mind naturally becomes clearer and more creative. The body becomes healthier and more energetic. And our thoughts, feelings, and actions gain spontaneous attunement with this evolutionary power of natural law.

Does it sound a bit abstract? It's actually a concrete experience and very practical for daily life. Here are a few perspectives:

A.J. Rachele, President of Technical Recruiters, an executive search firm headquartered in Washington, D.C.:

"Something very profound has taken place in my life since starting TM. I find that life is easier. It isn't so much of a struggle anymore.

"I've always noticed that there seemed to be a certain flow in nature, a flow to life. I could either fight against it—and meet with a lot of obstacles—or go with it and use it to my advantage.

"I find TM puts me in 'sync' with that flow in nature. I have much more energy and vitality now than I ever thought was possible. My ideas are more creative and timely and I seem to get more accomplished with far less effort."

Candace Martin, a Cincinnati attorney:

"Since I started TM, I find I'm in the right place at the right time much more often now, and my desires are more quickly fulfilled. I used to feel I was swimming upstream in my personal and professional life. Now I feel that events are going my way much more often. Life supported by natural law is a much better way to live."

Alliance with Natural Law

Why do individuals violate the laws of nature?

As Maharishi has said, education is responsible. "No educational system in the world is capable of training an individual to function spontaneously in accord with natural law. This lack in education is the cause of all problems in every area of life."

The solution to all problems then, as Maharishi has said, is spontaneous alliance with natural law.

Why?

Because when you closely examine them, all problems in life originate from the violation of natural law. It is violation of natural law that causes stress. Stress in an individual's life is the cause of sickness and suffering, and the build-up of stress among all the individuals in the world is the cause of war.

On the other hand, life spontaneously lived in accord with natural law is the basis for unrestricted and all-fulfilling progress for the individual, and the foundation for lasting peace and prosperity for the whole of mankind.

CHAPTER 6

Creating World Peace

W orld peace is the personal and immediate requirement of every significant individual in the world today, and it must be fulfilled today, without waiting for tomorrow."

—Maharishi

Consider the Problem of War

• Since 1,000 B.C. there have been over 8,000 major peace treaties ending wars or preventing new ones. Each treaty lasted an average of no more than nine years.

• The League of Nations was founded in 1920 to ensure that "the Great War was the war to end war." Twenty years later World War II erupted.

• The United Nations was established in 1945 to end war once and for all. Since then there have been over 150 major wars.

Consider the Origin

The quest for peace has always been considered to be the responsibility of governments. Yet all means available to governments—treaties, negotiations, and agreements—have been tried and failed. Now with the onset of terrorism and the threat of nuclear war escalating in the world, it is neither wise—nor safe—to assume that they ever will.

What is the origin of war? And why have negotiations, etc. failed to deliver peace?

Maharishi explains: "War is just the outburst of the build-up of stress in the world which is the result of all the individuals in society continually violating the laws of nature.

"Government, therefore, has been incapable of creating peace. This is because a government is not independent; it depends upon the collective consciousness of the individuals of the nation.

"As long as individuals continue to violate the laws of nature, they will continue to create stress in the collective consciousness of the nation. As a result, government trends and tendencies will be strained, and the world will face violence and conflict everywhere. World peace will only remain an abstract, unattainable idea."

Now consider the solution.

Individual Peace— The Basis of World Peace

"For the forest to be green, every tree must be green" is an old adage. The individual is the basic unit of world peace. For the world to be at peace, every individual must be at peace.

What is the basis of individual peace?

Maharishi: "Happiness is the basis of peace. Unless an individual is happy, any sense of peace he may have will be constantly disturbed. To enjoy real, lasting happiness an individual must enjoy increasing satisfaction and contentment in life. For this he must grow in energy, creativity, and intelligence day by day.

"The unified field is a field of infinite dynamism, an unlimited reservoir of energy and intelligence. It is the source of all the laws of nature that promote the orderly progress of life everywhere.

"The experience of the unified field gained during TM brings life into accord with this evolutionary power of nature. It promotes unrestricted and fulfilling progress for the individual—the basis of increasing happiness in life. And happiness alone can structure a permanent state of peace."

Foundation for World Peace

According to the scientific research, TM reduces stress, improves health, increases creativity and intelligence, increases productivity, improves relationships, and promotes the progress and happiness of the individual. It aligns life with the evolutionary force of natural law and can therefore be seen to provide the essential foundation for world peace—a peaceful individual.

("But that would mean that everyone in the world would have to practice TM to create peace," you say. "Is that a practical approach to world peace?")

Actually, there is a more practical solution:

Scientific research conducted during the past decade has shown that a small number of people practicing TM in any country is sufficient to produce a powerful influence of the evolutionary power of natural law and thereby create peace in the world.

The approach is a new one, but the research is impressive and the effect can be easily understood from recent discoveries in modern physics.

One Percent for World Peace

In 1960, just three years after founding the TM movement, Maharishi made a prediction. He said that if one percent of the world's population practiced Transcendental Meditation there would be no more wars.

At that time, there were too few meditators in the world for scientists to test the prediction, even on a small scale.

But by the end of 1974, over 250,000 people were meditating in the United States, and many small cities in the country even had one percent of their population practicing the TM technique.

The first scientific research to test Maharishi's prediction occurred in December 1974, when researchers measured quality-of-life indicators in four cities where one percent of the population was practicing the TM technique. Such standard and publicly accessible indices as crime statistics, accident rates, and hospital admissions were examined.

Decreased Crime in One Percent Cities

When these findings were compared with similar research from four control cities matched for population density, geography, economic conditions, etc., a remarkable discovery was made:

The cities with one percent of their populations practicing the TM program showed a decrease in crime rate while the matched control cities showed an increase in crime rate (as did the U.S. as a whole).

The researchers then expanded their study to include 11 one percent cities and 11 control cities. Their findings: a 16.6 percent reduction in crime rates among the one percent cities compared to the non one percent cities.

What did it mean?

It was the first scientific validation of his 1960 prediction that the quality of life could be improved through a small percentage of a population practicing TM.

Maharishi said: "With one percent of a city's population practicing TM, crime rates decrease. One percent of the world's population practicing the TM program will neutralize stress and negativity, and promote positivity and peace throughout the world. With just this first scientific research on the sociological effects of TM we can see the onset of a new age of progress and harmony for all mankind."

On January 12, 1975, in the presence of eminent scientists, educators, business leaders, and the world press, Maharishi inaugurated the dawn of the Age of Enlightenment for the world.

TM Is the Causal Factor

The sociological research increased. The 11-city study was expanded yet again to include 48 cities, with similar results. Entitled, "The Transcendental Meditation Program and Crime Rate Change in a Sample of Forty-Eight Cities," the research paper was published in the *Journal of Crime and Justice* (Vol. IV, 1981).

Since 1974, TM crime rate studies have been conducted in hundreds of cities in the United States using some of the most sophisticated, computerized, statistical procedures to control for a broad spectrum of variables.

The conclusion: TM program participation was seen to be the causal factor in crime rate reductions in cities and metropolitan areas throughout the nation. Scientists named the effect the "Maharishi Effect."

"Is this possible?" you ask.
Yes, and we'll discuss how in a moment.

The TM-Sidhi Program

Concurrent with all of this, a new development was taking place that was to have a profound impact on the direction of TM research.

In 1976, Maharishi introduced the TM-Sidhi program, which he described as advanced procedures or natural extensions of the TM program "to train consciousness to function from the unified field of natural law, the self-referral state of pure consciousness."

Maharishi explained that the TM-Sidhi program trained the awareness to function in the same self-interacting style as the intelligence of nature. In this way, Maharishi said, the individual would gain the support of the total potential of nature's creativity and intelligence for the fulfillment of his desires in daily life.

Scientific research showed that the TM-Sidhi program significantly enhanced the benefits of the TM technique. It increased brain wave coherence, as well as increased creativity and intelligence, and promoted longevity.

Most dramatically, sociological research

showed that the practice of the TM-Sidhi program by a small number of people together in one place had a very powerful effect on society as a whole—even more powerful than the one percent TM effect.

It was found that only the square root of one percent of a population practicing the TM-Sidhi program together in one place was required to create an influence of order and coherence in the entire population.

"But how is all of this possible?" you ask. "How can people meditating alone in their homes or offices, or together in a group, influence other people across town—or across the country—who aren't even meditating?"

Good question.

Super Radiance Effect:
Action-at-a-Distance

Two corks are floating in a sink of water six inches apart. Push down one cork, release it, and the other cork bobs up-and-down.

Driving to the grocery store, you turn on the radio. A disc jockey plays a record 50 miles away. The music fills your car.

These are examples where one object can influence another object at a distance. In physics, this phenomenon is called "action-at-a-distance."

How does it happen?

Through the influence of waves traveling through an underlying field. Water links the two corks, and the electromagnetic field links radio station and car radio.

Connecting all matter in the universe are unseen, fundamental fields—the electromagnetic field, the gravitational field, and the fields of the weak and strong forces binding the center of the atom.

At their basis, according to supersymmetric unified field theories, is the unified field, which creates and connects everything in the universe together—all fields, all matter, everything, everybody.

The Behavior of Fields

One interesting characteristic about the behavior of fields is the manner in which waves travel through them.

For example, consider the ordinary light radiating from your reading lamp. It is the product of innumerable light waves that are random and incoherent in their pattern. Take any 100 of these incoherent light waves and they produce the light of 100 separate light waves. Because of this the light from your lamp is bright enough for you to read the book in your lap but not nearly bright enough, say, to reach the moon.

On the other hand, if those random light waves are made coherent so that the peaks and valleys of each wave are in step with each other, then the total power of the light waves becomes far greater than when they function separately. Their power becomes the square of the actual number of waves. Take those 100 light waves again, make them function coherently together, and they will produce a light as bright as 10,000 individual light waves.

This coherent light is called laser light. It can be bounced off the moon, used to conduct surgery, or used to play a laser disc recording. This phenomenon has been called the "superradiance effect."

The Field Effects of Consciousness

How, then, can a small number of experts in the Transcendental Meditation and TM-Sidhi program affect a large population—at a distance?

Scientists said it could happen only if consciousness, experienced in its self-referral state during TM, is a field, and only if it is the same unified field that underlies all of nature.

They said that only a field can produce the influence of "action-at-a-distance," and only the unified field would be able to account for the wide-ranging effects on society observed with the collective practice of the TM and TM-Sidhi program. This is because on the level of the unified field everything in nature is connected.

The scientists predicted that if a group of experts in the TM and TM-Sidhi program could, in fact, produce an influence of coherence on the level of the unified field, then, according to the behavior of fields, that coherence would spread throughout the environment to less coherent places.

That's the hypothesis.

Now does it actually happen? What is the evidence? And how can it be measured?

Measuring the Trends of Time

In the past decade scientists have developed sophisticated statistical procedures to analyze changing trends in society. These methods are helpful to researchers attempting to determine why these changes occur.

For example, sickness rates might be found to be suddenly decreasing in a particular city. Why? Is it due to a public health program recently introduced into the school system, or is it simply a seasonal change?

Through these advanced statistical procedures, scientists are better able to identify the reason (or reasons) for the decrease in sickness rates in the city, eliminate alternative explanations, and hopefully produce the same effect again, perhaps on a wider scale.

TM Effects on Quality of Life

Extensive scientific research, employing many of these statistical procedures, have been conducted throughout the world to gauge the effects of the Transcendental Meditation and TM-Sidhi program on the quality of life in society.

The research has demonstrated repeatedly that when the square root of one percent of a population practices the TM and TM-Sidhi program together in one place there are marked decreases in negative tendencies such as crime, sickness, and accident rates, as well as instances of turbulence and violence in society. The research has also shown significant increases in positive trends, such as improvements in economic conditions.

(Note: Copies of all of the original research articles on the Transcendental Meditation technique are available through the International Center for Scientific Research, Maharishi International University, Fairfield, Iowa, 52556.)

7,000 Assembly at MIU

The largest of these experiments occurred from December 17, 1983, to January 6, 1984, at Maharishi International University in Fairfield, Iowa.

Seven thousand experts in the TM and TM-Sidhi program from over 50 nations gathered at MIU to create "an upsurge of coherence" for the whole world. Seven thousand is approximately the square root of one percent of the world's population.

The findings? The results included an immediate increase in positivity in situations of international conflict and a dramatic rise in the world stock index—the compilation of the 19 major stock markets. (Social scientists consider the stock index to be a sensitive barometer of the national mood and the confidence of the people in their economy.)

Available data from major countries on several continents also showed that traffic fatalities per miles driven and the incidence of infectious diseases dropped during the assembly, while patent applications and other signs of creativity and positivity rose.

And after the assembly? All the positive trends returned to the usual patterns that had characterized them prior to the assembly.

A New Formula for Peace

Based on these findings, as well as similar results from several other large assemblies held throughout the world, Maharishi declared 1987 to be the Year of World Peace. And he presented his program to create world peace, which included a plan to establish a permanent group of 7,000 experts collectively practicing the Maharishi Technology of the Unified Field together in one place.

Maharishi explained that the group of experts will "create an indomitable influence of coherence and positivity in world consciousness to ensure that all political, religious, social, and economic trends in the world will always remain positive and enriching."

For There to Be Peace in Society...

Maharishi also laid out a plan whereby every individual can contribute his or her share to promote peace:

"For there to be peace in society, there must be peace in the individuals in society. TM is a technique for gaining peace. If you have peace then you should engage in creating world peace by bringing your friends and family to start this practice. Unless you create peace in your family and friends, your own peace will be fragile and world peace will have no meaning for you. With peace in every home in our precious family of nations, heaven will descend on earth."

The following charts represent a few of the research studies conducted on the collective effects of the TM and TM-Sidhi program for society.

IMPROVED QUALITY OF LIFE IN U.S. CITIES

DECREASED CRIME

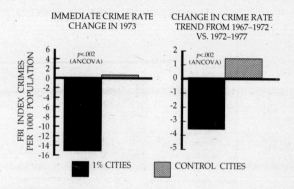

The results show that cities in which one percent of the population had been instructed in the Transcendental Meditation program by 1972 displayed decreased crime rate during the next year (1973) and decreased crime rate trend during subsequent years (1972-1977) in comparison to 1967-1972 in contrast to control cities matched for geographic region, population, college population, and crime rate.

M.C. Dillbeck, G. Landrith, D. Orme-Johnson, "The Transcendental Meditation Program and Crime Rate Change in a Sample of Forty-Eight Cities," *Journal of Crime and Justice* 4 (U.S.A.: 1981): 25-45.

IMPROVED QUALITY OF LIFE IN A STATE OF THE U.S.

IMPROVEMENTS IN RHODE ISLAND

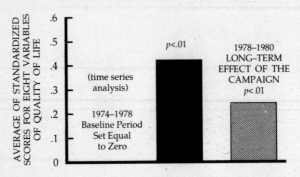

THREE–MONTH "IDEAL SOCIETY CAMPAIGN"

A prospective study was performed to assess the effects of the group practice of the TM and TM-Sidhi program on the quality of life in Rhode Island. The number of TM-Sidhi program participants was sufficient to create the Maharishi Effect for the entire state. A time-series analysis was performed on a monthly index that assessed the quality of life in Rhode Island in comparison to a control state. The index was comprised of the following variables: crime rate, motor vehicle fatality rate, cigarette consumption rate, auto accident rate, death rate (other than due to motor vehicles), alcoholic beverage consumption, unemployment rate, and pollution (suspended particulates). During the experimental period, there was a significant improvement in the quality of life in the state of Rhode Island.

M.C. Dillbeck, K.L. Cavanaugh, T. Glen, D.W. Orme-Johnson, and V. Mittlefehldt, "Consciousness as a Field: The Transcendental Meditation and TM-Sidhi Program and Changes in Social Indicators," *The Journal of Mind and Behavior* 8 (USA: 1987): 67-103.

REDUCED VIOLENCE
IN LEBANON

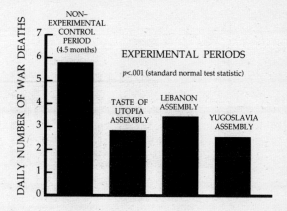

Time-series impact assessment analysis over a six-month period of the Lebanon war indicated that during the three experimental periods of collective practice of the Transcendental Meditation and TM-Sidhi program, there was a 50 percent reduction in mean number of reported war deaths. (The data source was daily quantitative content analysis of Lebanese news sources—*Al Nahar, Al Anwar, Le Reveil,* and *L'Orient* in Beirut, Lebanon.)

D.W. Orme-Johnson, C.N. Alexander, J.L. Davies, "Peace Project in the Middle East: Effects of the Maharishi Technology of the Unified Field on Conflict and Quality of Life in Israel and Lebanon." Presented at the Midwest Psychological Association, Chicago, May, 1987.

IMPROVED ECONOMIC TRENDS

INCREASED WORLD INDEX OF INTERNATIONAL STOCK PRICES

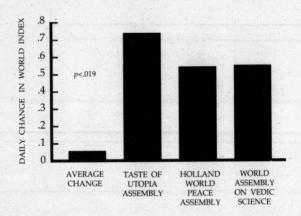

Based on previous research, scientists predicted in advance that three large international World Peace Assemblies would have a measurable positive influence on trends of life throughout the world. The number of experts practicing the Transcendental Meditation and TM-Sidhi program at these assemblies approached or surpassed 7,000—approximately the square root of one percent of the world's population—a figure which prior studies had discovered to be sufficient to influence an entire population. Time-series analysis showed that during the three experimental periods, the World Index of International Stock Prices (an arithmetic average weighted by market value of the stock markets in 19 countries) increased significantly.

Reference I: M.C. Dillbeck and J. Davies, "Intervention Studies on Reduction of Domestic and International Violence through Collective Consciousness," presented at the Third Midwest Conference for the United States Institute of Peace, University of Minnesota, Minneapolis, Minn., May 23, 1987. Reference II: D.W. Orme-Johnson, "Conflict Resolution and Improved Quality of Life through the Maharishi Technology of the Unified Field," given as part of a presentation on Maharishi's Program to Create World Peace at Dag Hammarskjold Auditorium, United Nations, New York, N.Y., June 3, 1987.

DECREASED CONFLICT
DECREASED INTERNATIONAL CONFLICTS

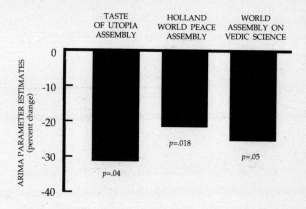

Time-series analysis of three large international World Peace Assemblies (see "Improved Economic Trends.") showed that significant reductions in international conflicts occurred globally during the three experimental periods. (Conflict was measured by blind content analysis of the *New York Times* for the Utopia and Vedic Science Assemblies and the *London Times* for the Holland Assembly). Time-series analysis also demonstrated decreases in auto fatalities and infectious diseases in the U.S.

Reference I: M.C. Dillbeck and J. Davies, "Intervention Studies on Reduction of Domestic and International Violence through Collective Consciousness," presented at the Third Midwest Conference for the United States Institute of Peace, University of Minnesota, Minneapolis, Minn., May 23, 1987. Reference II: D.W. Orme-Johnson, "Conflict Resolution and Improved Quality of Life through the Maharishi Technology of the Unified Field," given as part of a presentation on Maharishi's Program to Create World Peace at Dag Hammarskjold Auditorium, United Nations, New York, N.Y., June 3, 1987.

CHAPTER 7

The Next Step: How to Start

Why do people decide to start TM? *you ask.*
*Good question. People start TM for a wide
variety of reasons. Some may learn the technique
at the recomendation of their doctor to help treat
a specific stress-related problem, such as high
blood pressure. Others may be quite healthy but
decide to start because they want to use more of
their intelligence or enjoy greater inner happiness
in life. Others may start TM as a contribution to
world peace.*

*Whatever the reason—or reasons—why you
would decide to learn TM, with the regular practice of the technique, all of the overall positive
benefits to the mind, body, and behavior naturally develop. TM is one procedure which simultaneously strengthens all aspects of life. It's like
watering the root of a plant to nourish the entire
plant in one simple stroke.*

How do you learn it?
That's next.

Seven Steps to Learn TM

The Transcendental Meditation program is taught through a seven-step course of instruction in over 1,500 TM centers—called Capitals of the Age of Enlightenment—throughout the world.

The course includes two lectures, which provide the necessary intellectual understanding to start the technique, and four consecutive days of actual instruction—about two hours each day.

The structure is as follows:

Step 1—An Introductory Lecture

The first step is a public lecture which provides an introduction to the TM program and presents a vision of possibilities that result from the regular practice of the technique. The lecture lasts about 60 minutes and includes:

- Definition—what TM is and is not.
- Benefits—the scientifically validated effects of the technique for improving mental potential, health, and social behavior, and for promoting world peace.
- How to start the technique—an outline of the seven-step course of instruction to learn TM.

Step 2—A Preparatory Lecture

The second step is also a public lecture, which discusses the mechanics of the TM technique. It lasts about 90 minutes and includes a discussion of:

- How TM works.

• Why TM is easy to learn and effortless to practice.

• How TM is unique and different from all other techniques of meditation or self-development.

• The origin of the TM technique.

Step 3—A Personal Interview

The third step, a personal interview with a trained teacher of the TM technique, provides an opportunity to ask any additional questions you might still have and to make an appointment for personal instruction. The interview takes about 15 minutes.

Step 4—Personal TM Instruction

The fourth step is the actual instruction in the TM technique, which is held on a one-to-one basis with a qualified TM teacher. It is now that you'll learn the TM practice. Personal instruction takes about 90 minutes.

Step 5—First Day of Checking Seminar

The fifth step begins a 3-day series of checking seminars following personal instruction in TM. This step is held the day after your personal instruction. It is to review the mechanics of the TM technique and to verify and validate the correctness of your practice. This seminar is attended by all the other people who received personal TM instruction the previous day. This lasts about 90 minutes.

Step 6—Second Day of Checking Seminar

This sixth step is held on the second day after your personal instruction. It is to answer any new questions you might have, verify the correctness of your TM practice, and discuss the mechanics of stabilizing the benefits of the TM technique. This lasts about 90 minutes.

Step 7—Third Day of Checking Seminar

This seventh step is held on the third day after your personal instruction. It is to answer any new questions you might have, verify the correctness of your TM practice, and gain a vision of the goal of the TM program—the development of full human potential in higher states of consciousness. This lasts about 90 minutes.

Complete Follow-Up Program

After these seven steps of TM instruction, there is a complete follow-up program which is available on an optional basis for every meditator. The program includes personal checking to ensure continued correctness of your practice, advanced lectures, seminars, residence courses, etc.

The seven steps, plus the follow-up program, are offered on a regular basis through TM centers in cities throughout the United States. (To find out the lecture and teaching schedule in your local area, contact the TM center nearest you by consulting the listing "Transcendental Meditation" in the white pages of your telephone book.)

Two Requirements to Learn

There are two very practical requirements to learn TM:

1) Time. You must have the time to learn TM properly, which means you must be able to attend Steps 4-7 of instruction on the four consecutive days that they are offered.

The introductory and preparatory lectures, as well as the personal interview with a TM teacher, can be attended at your convenience. However, the actual four days of instruction must be attended in their proper sequence over four consecutive days.

If, for example, you know that you will be out of town during one of the four days of instruction, then wait until the next course is offered so that you can attend all four days in a row.

2) A Course Fee. In the United States, the TM program is taught under the auspices of the World Plan Executive Council, a non-profit, tax-exempt, educational organization.

A course fee is requested at the time of your personal instruction, which is used to cover the salaries of the teachers and the administrative expenses of the organization. The course fee entitles you to the four days of instruction in the TM program from a trained TM teacher plus the on-going follow-up program.

The course fees for instruction in the TM program are: $75 for a high school student, $125 for a college student, $190 for a retired person, $390 for an adult, and $590 for a family. (Contact your local TM center to check for any possible changes in the course fee structure.)

Is TM Worth It?

Here are two perspectives:

"When someone asks me about TM, I always use an analogy. I ask them, 'If you could purchase a chair for a few hundred dollars that would be so comfortable that just by sitting in it for 15-20 minutes all of the stress and fatigue of the day would melt away, and you would feel a deep sense of happiness and peace, would you buy it?'

"'Of course,' they say.

"Then, I tell them, 'What if it weren't a chair at all, which will wear out or break down after a few years, but a simple technique that you can practice sitting in any chair and get those same benefits?'

"Then they really get interested.

"I tell them, 'That's what TM is, and that's what TM does for me—and everyone else I know who practices it. TM is the best investment I've ever made because it's been an investment in myself.'"

Catherine Lyons, 76
Grandmother
San Francisco

"When I started TM several years ago I was still in college and any expense was a major consideration. I found myself hesitant to start TM for that reason. But after thinking about it for a while, I realized that I was actually selling myself a bit short. Here was a technique with a scientific track record that I knew could reduce stress, improve my health, and give me more energy and creativity to help me accomplish all that I want in my life.

"What kind of value could I put on that? I started TM and the money has never been a factor in my mind since. The follow-up program has been great and I have access to TM centers around the world for the rest of my life. It's definitely worth it. Actually, looking back on it, I only wish I had started 10 years earlier than I did."

Charles Lieb
First Vice President
E.F. Hutton
Washington, D.C. Office

After This Book—
The Next Step

"What do I do next?" you ask.

What do you do now, after reading this book, if you're interested in starting TM—or if you simply want some more information about the technique?

The next step is to attend a preparatory lecture.

"But isn't the introductory lecture first?"

With the information presented in this book, you've gained most of the knowledge discussed in the introductory lecture. You can now go on to the second step, which is the preparatory lecture.

The preparatory lecture, as we mentioned earlier, provides you with a clear explanation of how TM actually works, how it is unique to all other systems of meditation and self-development, as well as gives you an understanding about the origin of the technique. You can contact your local TM center to find out the schedule of the free preparatory lectures in your area.

"And if I have some questions about material covered in this book?"

Again contact your local TM center and speak to a TM teacher. Or you can ask your questions at the preparatory lecture. All TM teachers have received extensive training—up to a year of study—to teach this simple, natural, yet very precise technique. They will be happy to answer all of your questions.

"One last question?"
Certainly.
"Is TM simple for *everyone* to learn?"
Yes.
"And you think I could practice it?"
Easily.

"Thank you very much."
Thank you.

CHAPTER 8

Questions & Answers

What does TM do?

TM provides your mind and body with the unique and profound state of restful alertness. The body gains an extraordinarily deep state of rest while the mind settles down to a state of inner calm and wakefulness. This process dissolves deeply-rooted stress and tension, rejuvenates the entire system, infuses the mind with creativity and intelligence, and provides the basis for dynamic, successful activity.

I play tennis to relax. A friend of mine jogs. Doesn't exercise do the same thing as TM?

No. Tennis, jogging, a fishing trip, golf, gardening, reading a book, soothing music, bowling, etc., are all relaxing, enjoyable activities. They provide a welcome change of pace, a break in the routine.

The question is: While they may seem relaxing, do they actually release deeply-rooted stress and tension? No.

This is because even though they may feel relaxing, nonetheless, they keep the mind and body engaged in activity.

What is nature's antidote to stress?

Very deep rest.

TM is unique. It is not just another form of activity or recreation. TM is a scientifically-validated technique for providing the entire system with very deep rest—the deepest, most natural rest possible.

This deep rest has been shown to release the accumulated stress and tension that nothing else comes close to eliminating—not a good night's sleep, a restful vacation, relaxation exercises, an invigorating tennis match, or a walk in the park.

Will TM lower my high blood pressure? And how long does it take to get all the benefits found by the research?

Scientific research shows that TM does reduce high systolic blood pressure. The research also shows that TM provides a wide range of other profound benefits for the mind, body, and behavior.

At the same time, the experience of teaching TM to over three million people throughout the world shows that the specific benefits of TM often vary from individual to individual. It's true that all those who practice TM notice positive growth and development in their life, nevertheless, it's not really possible to predict what particular benefits you might receive from the practice or even how long it will take before you would experience a specific benefit.

What has been shown by both the research and personal experience is that the correct practice of TM on a regular, twice daily basis is very important for gaining the most from the technique.

Is TM like hypnosis or other types of meditation techniques?

TM is unique.

Hypnosis involves suggestion. TM is natural and involves no suggestion. It is a simple procedure for providing the body with deep relaxation while the mind is settled and awake. Research shows that TM produces profound physiological changes during the technique—along with a wide range of benefits in activity—that completely distinguish it from hypnosis.

All other forms of meditation or self-development involve either concentration or contemplation. TM is easy to learn, effortless and enjoyable to practice, and involves neither concentration nor contemplation. Research comparing TM with other forms of meditation has shown TM to be twice as effective for reducing stress and anxiety.

Will TM make me so relaxed that I won't be motivated for success?

Just the opposite. By eliminating stress and tension, and increasing energy and intelligence, TM is the most practical basis for dynamism and success in life.

TM is like pulling an arrow back on a bow. Draw the arrow back two feet and the arrow flies forward 50 yards. TM naturally draws the mind back to its own source, a reservoir of energy, creativity, and intelligence. After 20 minutes of TM we plunge into activity refreshed and rejuvenated, with more creativity and intelligence.

The result: Do less and accomplish more—with greater energy, success, and satisfaction in all endeavors.

Is TM difficult to learn?

TM is easy to learn and effortless to practice. Over one million Americans—and three million people worldwide—of every age (10 years and up), profession, education, and religion have learned TM and enjoy its benefits.

Can I learn TM from a book or a tape?

No. Each person who learns TM is unique; each person has a different nervous system and therefore a different pace of learning. To ensure that you learn the technique properly requires personal instruction from a qualified TM teacher. Reading a book or listening to a tape cannot provide the experience of the profound state of restful alertness, nor can it anticipate or answer all of the questions each person might have while learning the practice. With proper personal instruction, you can enjoy the technique for life—as well as all of the benefits it naturally unfolds.

When I start TM do I have to join an organization?

No. Once you've learned TM you can practice the technique on your own. There is, however, a complete follow-up program, available to all meditators on an optional basis, to ensure that they continue to practice TM correctly and gain maximum benefits. You can take advantage of this program at your convenience.

Where do you meditate?

TM is practiced sitting comfortably with the eyes closed for 20 minutes twice a day. It can be done anywhere—at home, in your office, on an airplane, on a train going to work, on a camping trip. Anywhere.

And anyone can do it?

Yes. Anyone of any age, profession, religion, education, or culture.

It doesn't matter if you believe in TM or not. You can be 100 percent skeptical about the technique and it will still work perfectly.

And for those people who think,

"I could never sit still for 20 minutes," or—

"I'm too high strung, I could never relax," or—

"I'll probably be the first person in the world who won't be able to learn it..."

Don't worry.

Anyone can.

See for yourself.

About the Author

Robert Roth, 37, is a graduate of the University of California at Berkeley. He has been a teacher of the TM program since 1972, and has taught the TM technique to executives and employees in many of America's largest corporations, as well as to faculty and students in universities and schools throughout the country. He has also directed TM centers in Washington, D.C., San Francisco, Detroit, and Seattle. Mr. Roth was a contributer to *Celebrating the Dawn* (Morrow) and the new edition of *The TM Book* (Fairfield Press).